HOME STRE... EXERCISES FOR SENIORS

The Ultimate Guide To Unlock Your Body's Potential and Live Your Best Life with Easy-to-Follow Exercises, Designed Specifically for the Golden Years.

Teresa S. Nichols

1

Table of Content

Introduction

Mrs. Smith had always been a physically active person, but as she aged, she began to have joint problems. She was aware of the value of exercise but wasn't sure what activities were risk-free for elders like her. At the neighbourhood library, she once discovered a book called "Home Stretch Exercises for Seniors."

Mrs. Smith borrowed the book and started reading it at home eager to learn more about how she could be active while staying safe. She was happy to find that the book was simple to read and that it provided detailed directions and illustrations for numerous stretches that she could perform at home.

Due to stiffness in her neck and shoulders, Mrs. Smith made the decision to start with the upper body stretches. Her body and breathing were both under her control as she carefully followed the directions. After only a few days of completing the exercises, she was surprised to feel a substantial increase in her range of motion and flexibility.

Encouraged by this achievement, Mrs. Smith made the decision to attempt some of the lower body stretches as well. For releasing the stiffness in her hips and lower back, she discovered that the hamstring stretch was really beneficial.

The more Mrs. Smith incorporated the stretches into her daily regimen, the more she noticed additional advantages. She experienced an increase in energy and a decrease in daytime weariness. She even observed that her nighttime sleep was improving.

Overall, Mrs. Smith was ecstatic with the outcomes of using the book on senior stretching exercises at home. She was happy that as she grew older, she had discovered a reliable method for continuing to be physically active and healthy.

Stretching exercises can significantly improve how comfortable senior citizens feel in their bodies. As we get older, our mobility declines and stiffness may develop. Stretching regularly can assist in addressing these problems and enhancing general health and self-confidence.

It's never been simpler to feel flexible and invigorated, no matter your age, with our simple-to-do at-home stretch exercises for seniors! Thus, let's begin our road to greater health and energy.

Chapter 1 - Stretching: Overview

What is Stretching?

Stretching entails stretching and elongating the body's muscles and tendons as a kind of physical activity. Numerous techniques, such as static stretching, dynamic stretching, and PNF stretching, are available. Stretching can be done before or after exercise as a warm-up or cool-down activity or on its own.

Types of Stretching Exercises

Stretching exercises come in a wide variety, each with unique advantages and applications. Stretching exercises come in a variety of popular forms, including:

Static stretching

This entails maintaining a stretch in a still position for a while, typically for roughly 30 seconds. After exercise, static stretching is frequently performed to aid in muscle cooling and safeguard against harm. Static stretches include holding a quad stretch, touching your toes, and stretching your hamstrings while seated on the floor.

Dynamic stretching

Before exercising, this entails putting the muscles and joints through a range of motion, such as swinging the arms or legs. Dynamic stretching aids in warming up and preparing the body for exercise. Arm circles, high knees, and walking lunges are examples of dynamic stretching practices.

PNF stretching

Proprioceptive neuromuscular facilitation, or PNF, is the contraction and relaxation of muscles while stretching. Stretching in this way helps increase range of motion and flexibility. An illustration of PNF stretching would be to first stretch your hamstring, then compress the muscle by pressing your foot into the hand of a partner for a short period of time, before relaxing and extending the stretch even further.

Active stretching

This entails stretching the muscles directly, as by elevating the leg to release the hamstring. Active stretching helps to increase strength while also enhancing flexibility and mobility. Arm circles, trunk rotations, and leg swings are a few examples of active stretching.

Passive stretching

This entails extending the muscles by using an outside force, such a partner or a stretching tool. For a deeper stretch and increased flexibility, passive stretching is helpful. Passive stretching techniques include utilizing a yoga strap to extend your shoulders or doing hamstring stretches with a partner.

It's important to take your level of fitness and specific goals into account when including stretching into your routine. It's advisable to begin with gentle stretches if you're new to stretching and gradually increase the length and intensity of your stretching over time. Always warm up before stretching, hold each stretch for around 30 seconds, and steer clear of any uncomfortable positions.

Importance of stretching for seniors

Any fitness program must include stretching, and as we become older, this role only grows. As we age, our muscles and joints stiffen, and our flexibility and range of motion inevitably decline. This may result in a number of health problems, including diminished mobility, an elevated risk of falling, and a lower standard of living.

Seniors might benefit from stretching exercises to maintain and increase their range of motion, mobility, and flexibility. Stretching can also assist to lower the risk of injury, ease pain and stiffness in the muscles and joints, boost circulation, and enhance balance.

Stretching can benefit mental health as well, lowering tension and anxiety and enhancing general wellbeing. Seniors can benefit from greater physical and mental health benefits, leading to a higher quality of life, by including stretching activities in their daily regimen.

Stretching is also a low-impact exercise that seniors may do at home without any special equipment, making it a practical and accessible choice.

Stretching must always be done securely and within one's physical limitations, it should be noted. Before beginning any new fitness program, seniors should speak with their healthcare physician. To lower the chance of injury, they should always warm up properly before stretching.

Benefits of stretching exercises

The following are some major advantages of stretching exercises for seniors:

Increased range of motion and flexibility: As we become older, our muscles gradually stiffen up and lose some of their flexibility. Stretching exercises on a regular basis can assist to maintain and enhance flexibility, which can make it simpler to carry out daily tasks like walking, bending, and reaching.

Reduced chance of falling and getting hurt: Seniors are more likely to fall and get hurt when their balance and coordination are off. Exercises that stretch the muscles can assist to increase balance, coordination, and reaction time, which lowers the chance of falls and accidents.

Reduced stiffness and discomfort: As we age, our muscles and joints become more prone to stiffness and pain. By increasing blood flow to the muscles and joints, lowering inflammation, and releasing tension, stretching exercises can assist to relieve these symptoms.

Better posture: Back discomfort and decreased mobility are only two health problems that can be brought on by poor posture. Through the stretching of contracted muscles and the redressing of imbalances, stretching exercises can help to improve posture.

Improved circulation: Circulation is improved through stretching exercises, which can also lower the risk of cardiovascular disease by increasing blood flow to the muscles and joints.

Reduced anxiety and stress: Stretching exercises can have a relaxing impact on the body and mind, lowering stress and anxiety and enhancing general wellbeing.

Increased vitality and energy: An increase in energy and vitality can make it simpler to carry out everyday tasks and maintain an active lifestyle. Regular stretching exercises might help with this.

Safety Considerations

While stretching exercises can be a secure and efficient approach for seniors to increase their range of motion and flexibility, it's crucial to keep some safety precautions in mind to avoid harm. For seniors stretching at home, the following safety advice is provided:

Consult a healthcare professional: Seniors should speak with their healthcare practitioner before beginning any new fitness regimen to be sure they are physically capable of carrying out the activities safely.

Start out slowly: Seniors should begin their stretching activities with easy stretches and gradually build up to more strenuous poses that last longer. This will help to prevent injury and avoid overexertion.

Warm up properly: Seniors should warm up their muscles by engaging in light aerobic activity, such as walking or cycling, for at least 5 to 10 minutes before beginning any stretching activities. This will lessen the chance of damage and assist the muscles get ready for stretching.

Use good form: Seniors who practice stretching exercises should do it with good form to prevent overstretching their muscles and joints. Props like yoga blocks or straps may be used in this scenario to support the body and guarantee perfect posture.

Avoid bouncing: Seniors should refrain from bouncing or jerking motions during stretching exercises because these actions might harm the muscles and joints and put undue strain on them. Instead, stretches should be performed 2-4 times while being held for 15–30 seconds.

Listen to your body: Seniors should pay attention to their bodies and refrain from pushing themselves above their physical limits. They should cease stretching right once and seek medical advice if it hurts or feels unpleasant.

Stay Hydrated: Prevent muscle cramps and exhaustion by staying hydrated by drinking plenty of water prior to, during, and after stretching exercises.

Chapter 2 - Upper Body Stretches

Stretching exercises that focus on the arms, shoulders, neck, and upper back are known as upper body stretches. They are crucial for preserving these areas' flexibility and mobility, which can lower the risk of injury and enhance physical performance. Here are several stretches for the upper body that seniors can perform at home:

Shoulder roll

Shoulder rolls are a quick and efficient exercise that helps enhance shoulder mobility and ease neck and shoulder stress in seniors. How to do shoulder rolls is as follows:

- While standing or sitting, straighten your back and keep your arms at your sides.

- Tensing your neck and shoulder muscles, slowly elevate your shoulders near your ears.

- Hold for a short while before slowly rolling your shoulders back and down while pressing your shoulder blades together.

- Roll your shoulders in a smooth circular motion as you do so, moving them forward and up, then back and down.

- Repeat for 10-15 times, then reverse the shoulder rolls' direction and go through another 10-15 times.

- Throughout the workout, take deep breaths, inhaling as you lift your shoulders and exhaling as you lower them.

Shoulder rolls can be performed separately or as a warm-up exercise before performing other upper body exercises. By performing smaller or slower shoulder rolls for those with restricted mobility or shoulder pain, they can be adjusted to fit individual needs and abilities.

Tricep stretch

Seniors can increase their arm flexibility and range of motion with triceps stretches. The muscle that straightens the arm is called the triceps, and it is found near the back of the upper arm. Here's how to stretch your triceps:

- One arm should be raised straight up in the air while standing with your feet shoulder-width apart.

- To touch the centre of your back, bend your elbow and place your hand behind your head.

- By gently pulling back on your elbow with your other hand, you can extend your triceps muscle.

- Repeat on the opposite side after releasing the stretch after 15 to 30 seconds.

- Throughout the workout, take slow, deep breaths, inhaling as you stretch and exhaling as you relax.

Seniors can perform this stretch while seated if they put one hand behind their head and use the other to gently press their elbow back. Triceps stretches can be performed separately or in conjunction with other upper body stretches.

Chest stretch

An easy exercise that might help seniors with posture and stiffness in the upper body is the chest stretch. Here is the chest stretch technique:

- Straighten your back whether standing or sitting, and keep your shoulders loose.

- Palms facing in, clench your hands together behind your back.

- Squeezing your shoulder blades together, slowly raise your hands as high as you can.

- Release after 15–30 seconds of holding the stretch.

- Throughout the workout, take deep breaths, inhaling as you raise your arms and exhaling as you lower them.

Seniors can perform this stretch by squeezing through a doorway or a wall. Place your hands on the surface at shoulder height while standing with your back to the wall or doorway. When you begin to feel a stretch in your chest, slowly lean forward and hold the position for 15 to 30 seconds. Stretching your chest can be done separately or in conjunction with stretching your upper body.

Neck stretch

A gentle exercise called a neck stretch can assist seniors ease stress and stiffness in their shoulders and neck. Here's how to stretch your neck:

- Straighten your back while you stand or sit, and let your shoulders drop.

- Bring your ear nearer your shoulder as you slowly incline your head to one side.

- Feel a stretch on the opposite side of your neck as you slowly lower your head down toward your shoulder with your hand.

- Repeat on the opposite side after releasing the stretch after 15 to 30 seconds.

- While performing the exercise, take slow, deep breaths, breathing in as you tilt your head and breathing out as you release.

Seniors can perform this stretch by tilting or twisting their heads in either the forward or backward direction. A neck stretch can be performed on its own or as a component of a full-body stretching regimen. Seniors should cease performing neck stretches immediately and seek medical attention or physical therapy if they feel any pain or discomfort.

Upper back stretch

Seniors might benefit from upper back stretches to enhance their posture and release stress in their upper back and shoulders. Here are steps on how to stretch your upper back:

- Stand or sit with a straight back and your shoulders relaxed.

- With your elbows sticking out to the sides, rest your hands on the back of your head while interlacing your fingers.

- Bring your elbows together in front of your face while slowly contracting your shoulder blades.

- Release after 15–30 seconds of holding the stretch.

- Throughout the exercise, take deep breaths, inhaling as you grip your shoulder blades and exhaling as you let go.

Seniors can perform this stretch while standing with their arms outstretched in front of them, clasping their hands together and rounding their upper back, or while seated by placing their hands on the back of the chair and bending forward. The stretching of the upper back can be done separately or in conjunction with other upper body stretches.

Chapter 3 - Lower Body Stretches

Leg, hip, and lower back muscles are the focus of lower body stretches, a sort of stretching exercise. They are crucial for preserving these regions' flexibility and mobility, which may lower the risk of injury and enhance physical performance. Here are eight typical lower body stretches that older people may do at home:

Hamstring Stretch

The hamstring stretch is a simple yet efficient exercise for older citizens to increase their limb flexibility and mobility. Here's how to stretch your hamstrings:

- Sit on the floor with your legs straight in front of you.

- Reach for your toes while leaning forward gradually. Reach as far as you can while keeping your knees straight if you are unable to touch your toes.

- Release after 15–30 seconds of holding the stretch.

- As you do the exercise, take slow, deep breaths, inhaling as you stretch forward and exhaling as you release.

Seniors may do this stretch while standing and leaning forward with their hands on a table or chair for support, or while sitting on a chair with one leg extended in front of them and reaching for their toes. You may do hamstring stretches alone or as a part of a lower body stretching practice.

Quadriceps Stretch

Seniors might benefit from the quadriceps stretch to increase their thigh flexibility and mobility. Here's how to stretch your quadriceps:

- Your back should be straight as you stand with your feet hip-width apart.

- Bring your left heel toward your buttocks while bending your left knee.

- Holding onto a chair or wall for support if necessary, grip your left ankle with your left hand.

- Keep your hips forward and your knees close together.

- Repeat on the other side after releasing the stretch after 15 to 30 seconds.

- Throughout the exercise, take deep breaths, inhaling as you elevate your leg and exhaling as you let it go.

Seniors may do this stretch by laying on their side, pulling their heel toward their buttocks, or by utilizing a chair to help them stay balanced while gripping their ankle.

Stretching your quadriceps may be done alone or in conjunction with other lower body stretching exercises.

Hip Flexor Stretch

The hip flexor stretch is a useful exercise for older citizens to increase hip flexibility and mobility. Here's how to stretch your hip flexors:

- Kneel on the floor with one foot forward and the other foot firmly placed. Bend your knee at a 90-degree angle.

- Keep your back straight and your abdominals taut.

- Bring your hips forward as you slowly transfer your weight forward to feel the stretch at the front of your kneeling hip.

- Repeat on the other side after releasing the stretch after 15 to 30 seconds.

- Throughout the exercise, take slow, deep breaths, inhaling as you move your weight forward and exhaling as you let go.

Seniors may do this stretch standing up if they take a big step forward with one leg, bend that knee, and maintain the back leg straight with the foot firmly planted on the ground. Stretching your hip flexors may be done alone or in conjunction with other lower body stretching exercises.

Calf Stretch

The calf stretch is a quick yet effective exercise for seniors to increase their lower limb flexibility and mobility. Here's how to stretch your calves:

- Face the wall and place your hands on the wall at shoulder height.

- With your right leg, take a step back while maintaining a flat heel and a forward-pointing toe.

- Maintain a bent left knee and a flat left foot at all times.

- The stretch in your right calf will be felt when you lean forward and put your hands onto the wall.

- Repeat on the other side after releasing the stretch after 15 to 30 seconds.

- While doing the exercise, take slow, deep breaths, inhaling as you lean forward and exhaling as you release.

Seniors may do this stretch by putting their heel on a curb or step, letting their toes dangle, and hanging onto a wall or railing for support. You may do calf stretches alone or as part of a lower body stretching practice.

Ankle Stretch

An easy exercise that might help seniors increase the flexibility and mobility of their ankles is the ankle stretch. Here's how to stretch your ankles:

- Put your feet flat on the ground and relax on a chair.

- Pointing your toes forward, raise your right foot off the ground.

- Circumambulate your ankle slowly while moving your foot counterclockwise.

- After doing 5–10 revolutions in a single direction, switch and rotate your ankle counterclockwise.

- On the opposite foot, repeat the exercise.

Seniors may do this stretch while standing as well by putting one foot on a step or curb, letting the heel drop, and gently rotating the ankle in a circular manner. Ankle stretches may be performed alone or in conjunction with lower body stretches.

Chapter 4 - Core Stretches

Exercises known as "core stretches" concentrate on the muscles that make up the body's core, which are located in the hip, lower back, and abdominal regions. Stretching these muscles may lower the chance of injury while also improving flexibility, mobility, and posture. Seniors may benefit from core stretches by improving their stability and balance, which is vital as they age and become more prone to falling.

Spinal Twist

The muscles in the lower back, hips, and spine are the focus of the famous stretch known as the spinal twist. Seniors who wish to increase their flexibility, mobility, and balance can try this workout. Follow these steps to do a spinal twist:

- Sit on the ground with your legs out in front of you to start.

- Put your right foot on the ground outside of your left knee while bending your right knee.

- On the outside of your right knee, position your left elbow. To provide support, place your right hand on the ground behind you.

- Taking a deep breath, extend your spine. Turn your body to the right and glance over your right shoulder as you exhale.

- Breathe deeply while holding the stretch for 10 to 15 seconds.

- Repeat on the other side after letting go of the twist.

Seniors may extend their range of motion and improve the health of their spines by doing spinal twists. To avoid pushing your body above its limits, it's crucial to tackle this stretch cautiously.

Lower back Stretch

A simple yet powerful exercise that targets the lower back's muscles, the lower back stretch may help seniors gain more flexibility, mobility, and good posture. The steps to do a lower back stretch are as follows:

- Start by lying on your back with your knees bent and your feet flat on the ground.

- Take a big breath in and softly hug your knees to your chest as you exhale.

- Breathe deeply while holding the stretch for 10 to 15 seconds.

- Release the stretch, then do it again three to five times.

Seniors should proceed cautiously with this stretch and avoid pushing their bodies above their capacity. Seniors should cease the lower back stretch right away and talk with their doctor or physical therapist if they feel any pain or discomfort while practicing it.

Abdominal Stretch

An easy workout that targets the muscles in the belly, the abdominal stretch may help seniors gain better posture, flexibility, and core strength. The steps to do an abdominal stretch are as follows:

- Sit on the ground with your legs out in front of you to start.

- As you gently exhale, lean back and lay your hands on the ground behind you for support. Take a big breath in.

- Lift your feet off the floor and pull your knees to your chest while maintaining straight legs and a strong core.

- Breathe deeply while holding the stretch for 10 to 15 seconds.

- Release the stretch, then do it again three to five times.

Seniors should proceed cautiously with this stretch and avoid pushing their bodies above their capacity. Seniors should cease doing the abdominal stretch as soon as they feel any pain or discomfort and call their doctor or physical therapist right away.

Chapter 5 - Stretching Routines

Stretching routines are organized series of stretches intended to promote flexibility, mobility, and general physical well-being. They are targeted at certain body parts. These exercises, which may be done at home or in a gym, often include a range of stretches for various muscle groups, including the upper and lower body, the core, and the back.

Seniors' requirements and aspirations may be individually catered for, taking into consideration their age, degree of fitness, and any existing medical illnesses or injuries.

Warm-up Routine

A warm-up regimen consists of a series of easy exercises that are meant to get the body ready for more demanding physical activity.

A proper warm-up regimen progressively raises body temperature, speeds up heart rate, and gets the muscles, tendons, and joints ready for the motions needed in an exercise or activity.

Warm-up programs often include dynamic stretching exercises that emphasize movement and range of motion rather than holding static positions, as well as low-impact cardiovascular workouts like walking, running, or cycling. Exercises like walking lunges, leg swings, arm circles, and high knees are examples of dynamic stretching techniques.

A typical rule of thumb is to strive for 5–10 minutes of aerobic exercise followed by 5–10 minutes of dynamic stretching activities. However, the length of a warm-up regimen might vary depending on the intensity and duration of the following activity.

Warm-up exercises are crucial for seniors to avoid injury and prevent stress on their muscles and joints. Seniors may benefit from a suitable warm-up regimen by gradually increasing their intensity and endurance during physical exercise, which will enhance their general fitness and wellbeing.

Seniors should always proceed cautiously while doing warm-up exercises and get advice from their doctor or physical therapist before beginning any new fitness regimen. It's crucial to choose warm-up activities that are suitable for their level of fitness and to gradually raise the warm-up's intensity over time.

Full-body Routine

A full-body program is a thorough exercise schedule that concentrates on all the body's main muscle groups. This kind of fitness program often combines aerobic activities like jogging, cycling, or swimming with resistance training exercises like weight lifting or bodyweight exercises.

A full-body workout aims to improve physical fitness by enhancing strength, endurance, and flexibility. Exercises that target the chest, back, legs, arms, shoulders, and core muscles are part of a well-designed full-body regimen.

A full-body regimen may also incorporate stretching and mobility exercises to increase flexibility and range of motion in addition to strength training and aerobic workouts. Hip flexor stretches, calf stretches, and upper and lower back stretches are a few stretching exercises that may be included into a full-body regimen.

A full-body workout may help seniors in a variety of ways, both physically and mentally. For example, it can enhance muscular strength, bone density, balance, and coordination, as well as lower their chance of developing chronic illnesses like osteoporosis and heart disease. However, seniors should proceed with care while doing full-body exercises and speak with their doctor or physical therapist before beginning any new fitness regimen.

Seniors should choose exercises based on their current level of fitness, begin with modest weights or resistance bands, and gradually increase the intensity and length of the activity over time. To avoid strain or damage, it's also crucial to pay attention to the body and refrain from going over one's limitations

Targeted Routine

A focused or targeted program is a training schedule that concentrates on certain muscle groups or body parts. A focused regimen consists of exercises that isolate and develop certain muscles or muscle groups as opposed to working out the full body.

For instance, a specific fitness program for seniors can concentrate on leg and hip strengthening activities like lunges, squats, and leg presses to enhance balance and reduce falls. As an alternative, a focused regimen may concentrate on upper body movements like bicep curls and shoulder presses to strengthen the arms and shoulders.

Seniors who wish to address particular fitness objectives or areas of weakness might benefit from targeted workouts. To maintain total health and fitness, it's crucial to follow a balanced exercise regimen that incorporates activities for the whole body.

Seniors should speak with their doctor or physical therapist before beginning a targeted regimen to make sure the exercises are suitable for their level of fitness and any pre-existing medical concerns. To minimize injuries and maximize training benefits, it's crucial to do exercises with the correct form and technique.

Chapter 6 - Tips for Safe and Effective Stretching

Proper Form and Technique

When conducting stretching exercises, particularly for seniors, proper form and technique are essential. Stretching incorrectly might result in damage and perhaps exacerbate any underlying issues.

Maintaining good alignment is one of the most crucial components of proper form and technique when stretching. This entails maintaining a neutral posture and preventing overextension or body twisting. For instance, while doing a hamstring stretch, it's crucial to maintain a straight back and refrain from sloping the shoulders or bending at the waist.

Seniors should concentrate on breathing during stretching exercises in addition to good posture. The stretch will work better and there will be less chance of harm if you breathe properly. Seniors should take a deep breath before starting the stretch and let it out gently as they get into it.

Avoiding bouncing or jerking motions during stretching is a crucial component of appropriate form and technique. These motions increase the chance of injury and may strain muscles. Seniors should hold each stretch for 15 to 30 seconds, moving into and out of it gently and gracefully.

Seniors should choose stretching activities that are suitable for their level of fitness and any pre-existing medical issues. For example, seniors who have arthritis may need to alter some stretches to prevent placing strain on their joints.

Seniors should always undertake stretching exercises with good form and technique. Seniors should use care while stretching and get advice from their physician or physical therapist before beginning any new fitness regimen. Seniors may safely and efficiently increase their flexibility, range of motion, and general physical health by using the right form and technique.

Breathing Techniques

Stretching involves breathing, and using the right breathing methods may increase the health advantages of stretching activities. Seniors' entire physical health may be enhanced and their levels of stress reduced and increased with proper breathing techniques.

Senior citizens should concentrate on deep breathing when doing stretches. This entails taking a deep breath via your nose, filling your lungs with air, and then gently expelling through your mouth. Elderly people should try to breathe deeply into their abdomen rather than merely their chest.

Seniors may relax and prime their body for a stretch by taking a deep breath before starting. Seniors should softly exhale as they enter the stretch to ease any muscular tension. Seniors may stretch more deeply and boost the efficacy of their stretch by holding it for a short period of time while continuing to exhale.

Seniors might include meditation methods to their stretching regimen in addition to deep breathing. This may assist them in focusing on their breathing and calming their minds, which will help them unwind and reduce tension. Additionally, meditation may help seniors minimize their chance of developing chronic illnesses, strengthen their immune systems, and enhance their mental well-being.

Seniors must pay attention to their bodies and refrain from overstretching. While stretching, they should stop immediately and speak with their doctor or physical therapist if they feel any pain or discomfort. Seniors should check their comfort and level of relaxation before starting any stretching activities.

Alterations for Various Fitness Levels

Stretching exercises for seniors must be modified for individuals with varying degrees of fitness. Stretching exercises must be modified based on the flexibility and mobility of the senior since these factors might vary widely. Here are several adaptations for various levels of fitness:

Beginners: Seniors who have limited mobility or are new to stretching activities might begin with easy stretches that emphasize increasing flexibility and range of motion. They may also use supports to support their bodies while stretching, such as cushions, blankets, or yoga blocks. Neck stretches, shoulder rolls, and ankle stretches are a few examples of basic stretches.

Intermediate: Seniors who have been doing stretching exercises on a regular basis may advance to increasingly difficult stretches that call for more flexibility and balance. Lunges, spinal twists, and hamstring stretches are a few examples of intermediate stretches. To enhance the intensity, they may also attempt holding stretches for longer periods of time.

Advanced: Seniors with strong flexibility who routinely practice stretches may attempt increasingly difficult stretches that call for greater strength and balance. The split, backbends, and arm balances are a few examples of advanced stretches. To prevent damage, it's crucial to approach these stretches gently and cautiously.

People with reduced mobility: Stretching exercises may still be beneficial for seniors who have limited movement because of ongoing medical issues or accidents. To accommodate their constraints, they might adapt stretching exercises by sitting during leg stretches or utilizing a chair as support.

People who have arthritis: Seniors who have arthritis may adjust stretching activities by concentrating on mild range-of-motion exercises that concentrate on the damaged joints. To ease tight joints before stretching, they may also employ heat treatment, such as a warm compress or a hot bath.

Overall, it's critical to adapt stretching exercises to seniors' fitness levels in order to prevent injury and maximize benefits. Before beginning any new stretching regimen, seniors should speak with their doctor or physical therapist, particularly if they have any ongoing medical concerns or injuries.

Common Mistakes to Avoid

Stretching is a healthy practice that may enhance your range of motion, flexibility, and overall physical performance. However, there are certain frequent stretches errors that seniors do that might harm them or lessen the benefits of the exercise. Here are some frequent stretches errors to avoid:

Bouncing: During stretches, bouncing or jerking might cause damage or muscular strain. Stretching should be done gently and gradually without making any abrupt movements.

Overstretching: Holding a stretch for an extended period of time may potentially cause damage or muscular strain. Depending on their degree of fitness, seniors should hold stretches for a reasonable amount of time, often between 10 and 30 seconds.

Breathing too tightly: Holding your breath when stretching might cause the body to tense up and reduce the exercise's efficacy. Seniors who stretch should concentrate on calm, deep breathing to relax their muscles and increase oxygen flow.

Poor posture: Poor alignment from poor posture during stretches might result in injury. During stretches, seniors should maintain good alignment and form by keeping their shoulders relaxed and their spines straight.

Skipping warm-up activities: Skipping warm-up exercises might make stretching more risky for injury. Before stretching, seniors should warm up their muscles and joints to be ready for activity.

Ignoring discomfort: Ignoring pain when stretching may result in further harm or aggravate already present problems. Seniors should pay attention to their body and refrain from pushing themselves too far. Stretching should only be done if there are no pains or discomforts; otherwise, stop and visit a doctor.

Neglecting to stretch both sides of the body: This might result in muscular imbalances and lessen the efficacy of the workout. Stretching should be done on both sides of the body by seniors to encourage symmetry and balance.

Finally, seniors should be aware of these typical blunders and take precautions to prevent them while doing stretches. Seniors may benefit from stretching without running the risk of pain or discomfort by using appropriate form, avoiding rapid movements, and paying attention to their body.

Conclusion

Finally, stretching activities are a crucial part of a senior's healthy lifestyle. Stretching correctly may enhance your range of motion, flexibility, and overall physical performance. Seniors may maintain a healthy and active lifestyle by adding stretches for the upper body, lower body, and core into a program. To prevent injury and get the most out of stretching, pay close attention to good form, breathing methods, and adaptations for varied fitness levels. Seniors should also always listen to their body during stretching exercises and speak with their healthcare physician before starting any fitness regimen. Seniors may have more active and meaningful lives by including stretching on a regular basis in their regimen.

Encouragement to include stretching into their daily routine

I wish to exhort seniors to include stretching into their everyday routine. Stretching for only a few minutes a day may make a big difference in your physical health and wellness. Stretching may lower the risk of injury and enhance physical performance by enhancing flexibility, range of motion, and circulation.

Regular stretching may also aid elderly people in maintaining their independence and leading an active lifestyle. Balance and coordination may be enhanced, which are crucial for avoiding falls and preserving mobility. Stretching also helps elders manage arthritis and chronic pain by reducing muscular stiffness and stress.

Just keep in mind that stretching is not just for athletes and fitness fanatics. It is a quick and easy approach for seniors to keep themselves healthy and happy. I thus urge you to include stretching on a regular basis in your routine, whether you're trying to enhance your golf swing or just want to be able to tie your shoes more quickly. Start out slowly and build up the length and intensity of your stretches as you become more comfortable.

Before starting any workout regimen, pay attention to your body and speak with your doctor. You can reap the numerous advantages of stretching and keep up an active, healthy lifestyle for years to come with perseverance and consistency.

Dear Reader

Thank you for choosing to trust us by purchasing this book. Best wishes in your endeavours.

Teresa S. Nichols

Printed in Great Britain
by Amazon

43354989R00036